SPECIAL LEAN

AND GREEN

RECIPES

COLLECTION

Always a Different Meals Thanks to This Tasty
Cookbook

Carmen Bellisario

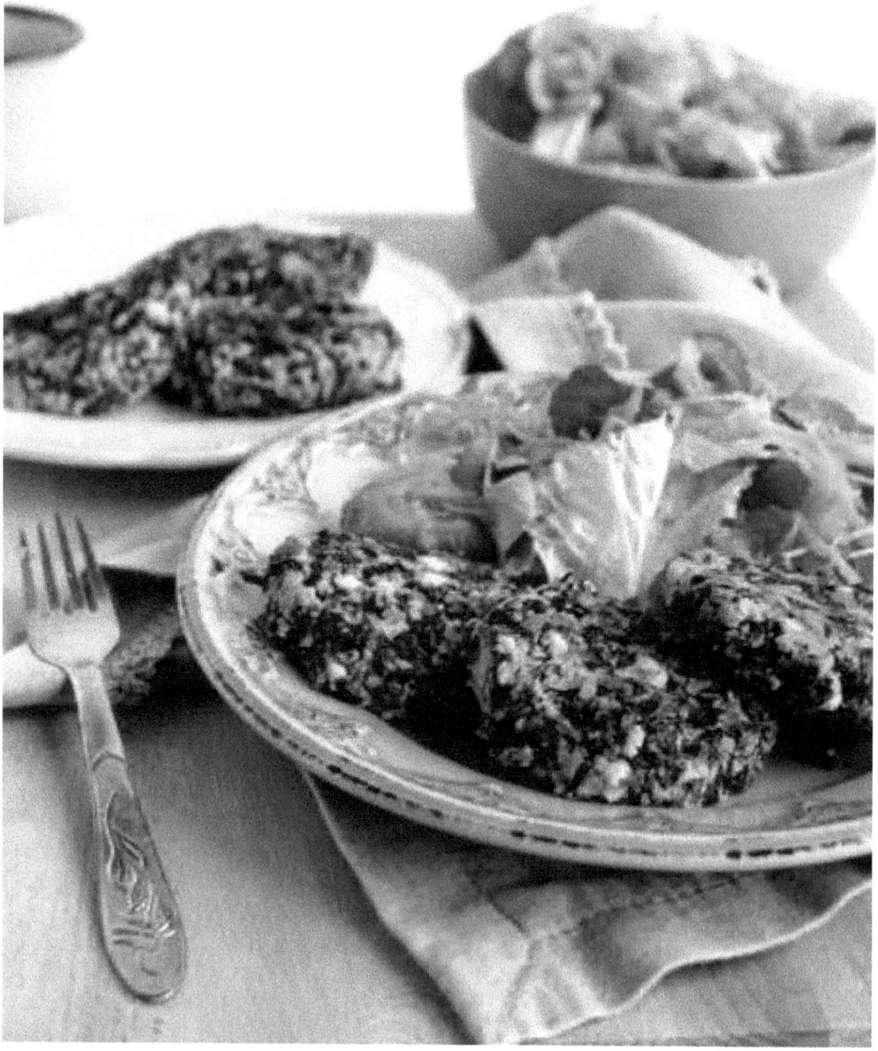

TABLE OF CONTENTS

Simple Beef Burgers

Servings: 4

Preparation time: 15 minutes

Cooking time: 10 minutes

Ingredients:

- 1-pound ground beef
- 1 large egg, lightly beaten
- ½ cup of seasoned breadcrumbs
- Salt and ground black pepper, as required
- 1 tablespoon of olive oil
- 6 cups of fresh spinach, torn
- 1 large tomato, chopped

Instructions:

1. Preheat the grill to medium heat.
2. Grease the grill grate.
3. In a large bowl, add the meat, egg, breadcrumbs, salt, black pepper and blend until well combined.
4. Make 4 (½-inch thick) patties from the mixture.

5. With your thumb, press a shallow indentation in the center of every patty.
6. Brush each side of every patty with oil.
7. Place the burgers onto the grill and cook, covered for about 4-5 minutes per side.
8. Serve alongside the spinach and tomato.

Beef & Spinach Burgers

Servings: 4

Preparation time: 15 minutes

Cooking time: 12 minutes

Ingredients:

For Burgers:

- 1-pound ground beef
- 1 cup of fresh baby spinach leaves, chopped
- ½ of small yellow onion, chopped
- ¼ cup of sun-dried tomatoes, chopped
- 1 egg, beaten
- ¼ cup of feta cheese, crumbled
- Salt and ground black pepper, as required
- 2 tablespoons of olive oil

For Serving:

- 3 cups of fresh spinach, torn
- 3 cups of lettuce, torn
- 2 tomatoes, sliced

Instructions:

1. For Burgers: in a large bowl, add all Ingredients apart from oil and blend until well combined.
2. Make 4 equal-sized patties from the mixture.
3. In a skillet, heat the oil over medium-high heat and cook the patties for about 5-6 minutes per side or until desired doneness.
4. Divide the lettuce, spinach, and tomato slices and onto serving plates.
5. Top each with 1 burger and serve.

Spicy Beef Burgers

Servings: 4

Preparation time: 20 minutes

Cooking time: 10 minutes

Ingredients:

For Burgers

- 1-pound lean ground beef
- ¼ cup of fresh parsley, chopped
- ¼ cup of fresh parsley, chopped
- ¼ cup of fresh cilantro, chopped
- 1 tablespoon of fresh ginger, chopped
- 1 teaspoon of ground cumin
- 1 teaspoon of ground coriander
- ½ teaspoon of ground cinnamon
- Salt and ground black pepper, as required

For Salad:

- 6 cup of fresh baby arugula
- 2 cups of cherry tomatoes, quartered
- 1 tablespoon of fresh lemon juice

- 1 tablespoon of extra-virgin olive oil

Instructions:

1. In a bowl, add the meat, ¼ cup of parsley, cilantro, ginger, spices, salt, and black pepper, and blend until well combined.
2. Make 4 equal-sized patties from the mixture.
3. Heat a greased grill pan over medium-high heat and cook the patties for about 3 minutes per side or until desired doneness.
4. Meanwhile, in a bowl, add arugula, tomatoes, juice, oil, and toss to coat well.
5. Divide the salad onto serving plates and top each with 1 patty.
6. Serve immediately.

Spiced Beef Meatballs

Servings: 4

Preparation time: 15 minutes

Cooking time: 20 minutes

Ingredients:

- 1-pound of ground beef
- 1 tablespoon of olive oil
- 1 teaspoon of dehydrated onion flakes, crushed
- ½ teaspoon of granulated garlic
- ½ teaspoon of ground cumin
- ½ teaspoon of red pepper flakes, crushed
- Salt, as required
- 6 cups of fresh baby spinach
- 1 cup of tomato, chopped

Instructions:

1. Preheat the oven to 400 degrees F.
2. Line a bigger baking sheet with parchment paper.
3. In a bowl, place all the Ingredients and with your hands, mix until well combined.
4. Shape the mixture into desired and equal-sized balls.

5. Arrange meatballs into the prepared baking sheet in a single layer and Bake for about 15-20 minutes or until done completely.
6. Serve hot alongside spinach and tomato.

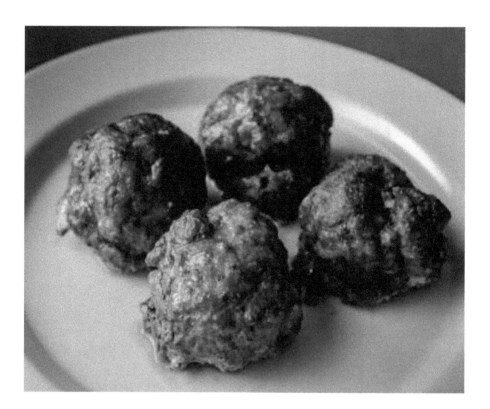

Beef & Veggie Meatballs

Servings: 6

Preparation time: 15 minutes

Cooking time: 30 minutes

Ingredients:

For Meatballs:

- ½ cup of carrot, peeled and grated
- ½ cup of zucchini, grated
- ½ cup of yellow squash, grated
- Salt, as required
- 1-pound lean ground beef
- 1 egg, beaten
- ¼ of a small onion, chopped finely
- 1 garlic clove, minced
- 2 tablespoons of mixed fresh herbs (parsley, basil, cilantro, chopped final

For Serving:

- 6 cups of fresh baby spinach
- 3 large tomatoes, sliced

Instructions:

1. Preheat your oven to 400 degrees F.
2. Line a large baking sheet with parchment paper.
3. In a large colander, place the carrot, zucchini and yellow squash and sprinkle with 2 pinches of salt. Put aside for at least 10 minutes.
4. Transfer the veggies over a towel and squeeze out all the moisture
5. In a large bowl, add squeezed vegetables, beef, egg, onion, garlic, herbs, salt, and blend until well combined.
6. Shape the mixture into equal-sized balls.
7. Arrange the meatballs onto the prepared baking sheet in a single layer.
8. Bake for about 25-30 minutes or until done completely.
9. Divide the spinach and tomato slices onto serving plates.
10. Top each plate with meatballs and serve.

Spicy Beef Koftas

Servings: 6

Preparation time: 15 minutes

Cooking time: 10 minutes

Ingredients:

- 1-pound ground beef
- 2 tablespoons of low-fat plain Greek yoghurt
- 2 tablespoons of yellow onion, grated
- 2 teaspoons of garlic, minced
- 2 tablespoons of fresh cilantro, minced
- 1 teaspoon of ground coriander
- 1 teaspoon of ground cumin
- 1 teaspoon of ground turmeric
- Salt and ground black pepper, as required
- 1 tablespoon of olive oil
- 8 cups of fresh salad greens

Instructions:

1. In a large bowl, add all the Ingredients apart from greens and blend until well combined.

2. Make 12 equal-sized oblong patties from the mixture.
3. In a large non-stick skillet, heat the oil over medium-high heat and cook the patties for about 10 minutes or until browned from each side, flipping occasionally.
4. Meanwhile, for sauce: In a bowl, add all the Ingredients and blend until well combined.
5. Serve the Koftas with the yoghurt sauce.

Beef Kabobs

Servings: 6

Preparation time: 15 minutes

Cooking time: 8 minutes

Ingredients:

- 3 garlic cloves, minced
- 1 tablespoon of fresh lemon zest, grated
- 2 teaspoons of fresh rosemary, minced
- 2 teaspoons of fresh parsley, minced
- 2 teaspoons of fresh oregano, minced
- 2 teaspoons of fresh thyme, minced
- 4 tablespoons of olive oil
- 2 tablespoons of fresh lemon juice
- Salt and ground black pepper, as required
- 2 pounds beef sirloin, cut into cubes
- 8 cups of fresh baby greens

Instructions:

1. In a bowl, add all the Ingredients except the meat and greens and blend well.

2. Add the meat and coat with the herb mixture generously.
3. Refrigerate to marinate for at least 20-30 minutes.
4. Preheat the grill to medium-high heat. Grease the grill grate.
5. Remove the meat cubes from the marinade and thread onto metal skewers.
6. Place the skewers onto the grill and cook for about 6-8 minutes, flipping after every 2 minutes.
7. Remove from the grill and place onto a platter for about 5 minutes before serving.
8. Serve alongside the greens.

Garlicky Beef Tenderloin

Servings: 19

Preparation time: 10 minutes

Cooking time: 50 minutes

Ingredients:

- 1 (3-pound) centre-cut beef tenderloin roast
- 4 garlic cloves, minced
- 1 tablespoon of fresh rosemary, minced
- Salt and ground black pepper, to taste
- 1 tablespoon of olive oil
- 15 cups of fresh spinach

Instructions:

1. Preheat your oven to 425 degrees F.
2. Grease a large shallow roasting pan.
3. Place the roast into the prepared roasting pan.
4. Rub the roast with garlic, rosemary, salt, and black pepper, and drizzle with oil.
5. Roast the meat for about 45-50 minutes.

6. Remove from oven and place the roast onto a chopping board for about 10 minutes.
7. With a knife, cut tenderloin into desired-sized slices and serve alongside the spinach.

Simple Steak

Servings: 4

Preparation time: 10 minutes

Cooking time: 10 minutes

Ingredients:

- 1 tablespoon of olive oil
- 4 (6-ounce of) flank steaks
- Salt and ground black pepper, to taste
- 6 cups of fresh salad greens

Instructions:

1. In a wok, heat the oil over medium-high heat and cook steaks with salt and black pepper for about 3-5 minutes per side.
2. Transfer the steaks onto serving plates and serve alongside the greens.

Rosemary Steak

Servings: 6

Preparation time: 15 minutes

Cooking time: 15 minutes

Ingredients:

- 3 garlic cloves, minced
- 2 tablespoons of fresh rosemary, chopped
- Salt and ground black pepper, as required
- 2 pounds flank steak, trimmed
- 8 cups of fresh baby kale

Instructions:

1. Preheat the grill to medium-high heat.
2. Grease the grill grate.
3. In a large bowl, add all the Ingredients except the steak and kale mix until well combined.
4. Add the steak and coat with the mixture generously.
5. Put aside for about 10 minutes.
6. Place the steak onto the grill and cook for about 12-15 minutes, flipping after every 3-4 minutes.

7. Remove from the grill and place the steak onto a chopping board for about 5 minutes.

8. Meanwhile, for sauce: in a bowl, add all the Ingredients and blend well.

9. With a pointy knife, cut the steak into desired sized slices.

10. Serve the steak slices alongside the kale.

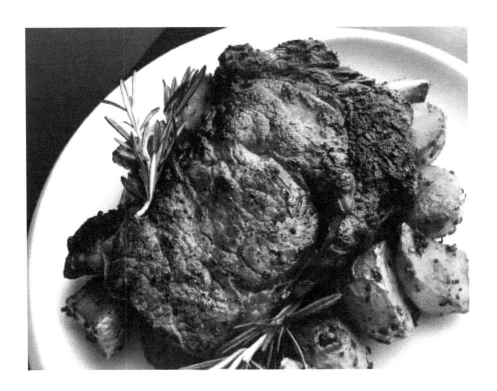

Spiced Flank Steak

Servings: 5

Preparation time: 10 minutes

Cooking time: 20 minutes

Ingredients:

- ½ teaspoon of dried thyme, crushed
- ½ teaspoon of dried oregano, crushed
- 1 teaspoon of red chili powder
- ½ teaspoon of ground cumin
- ¼ teaspoon of garlic powder
- Salt and ground black pepper, to taste
- 1½ pounds flank steak, trimmed
- 6 cups of salad greens

Instructions:

1. In a large bowl, add the dried herbs and spices and blend well.
2. Add the steaks and rub with mixture generously.
3. Put aside for about 15-20 minutes.
4. Preheat the grill to medium heat. Grease the grill grate.

5. Place the steak onto the grill over medium coals and cook for about 18–20 minutes, flipping once halfway through.
6. Remove the steak from grill and place onto a chopping board for about 10 minutes before slicing.
7. With a knife, cut the steak into desired sized slices and serve alongside the greens.

Simple Flank Steak

Servings: 4

Preparation time: 10 minutes

Cooking time: 8 minutes

Ingredients:

For Steak:

- 2 tablespoons of extra-virgin olive oil
- 4 (6-ounce of) flank steaks
- Salt and ground black pepper, to taste

For Salad:

- 6 cups of fresh baby arugula
- 3 tablespoons of extra-virgin olive oil
- 2 tablespoons of balsamic vinegar
- Salt and ground black pepper, to taste

Instructions:

1. In a sauté pan, heat the oil over medium-high heat and cook the steaks with salt and black pepper for about 3-4 minutes per side.

2. Meanwhile, For Salad: in a salad bowl, place all Ingredients and toss to coat well.
3. Divide the arugula onto serving plates and top each with 1 steak.
4. Serve immediately.

Steak with Green Beans

Servings: 2

Preparation time: 15 minutes

Cooking time: 10 minutes

Ingredients:

For Steak:

- 2 (5-ounce of) sirloin steaks, trimmed
- Salt and ground black pepper, as required
- 1 tablespoon of extra-virgin olive oil
- 1 garlic clove, minced

For Green Beans:

- ½ pound fresh green beans
- ½ tablespoon of olive oil
- ½ tablespoon of fresh lemon juice

Instructions:

1. For steak: Season the steaks with salt and black pepper evenly.

2. In a forged iron sauté pan, heat the vegetable oil over high heat and sauté garlic for about 15-20 seconds.

3. Add the steaks and cook for about 3 minutes per side.

4. Flip the steaks and cook for about 3-4 minutes or until the desired doneness, flipping once.

5. Meanwhile, for green beans: in a pan of boiling water, arrange a steamer basket.

6. Place the green beans in a steamer basket and steam covered for about 4-5 minutes.

7. Carefully transfer the beans into a bowl.

8. Add vegetable oil and juice and toss to coat well.

9. Divide green beans onto serving plates.

10. Top each with 1 steak and serve.

Veggie & Feta Stuffed Steak

Servings: 6

Preparation time: 15 minutes Cooking time: 35 minutes

Ingredients:

- 12 tablespoons of dried oregano leaves
- 1/3 cup of fresh lemon juice
- 2 tablespoons of olive oil
- 1 (2-pound) beef flank steak, pounded into ½-inch thickness.
- 1/3 cup of olive tapenade
- 1 cup of frozen chopped spinach, thawed and squeezed
- ¼ cup of feta cheese, crumbled
- 4 cups of fresh cherry tomatoes Salt, as required

Instructions:

1. In a large baking dish, add the oregano, juice and oil and blend well.
2. Add the steak and coat with the marinade generously.
3. Refrigerate to marinate for about 4 hours, flipping occasionally.

4. Preheat the oven to 425 degrees F.

5. Line a shallow baking dish with parchment paper.

6. Remove the steak from baking dish, reserving the remaining marinade in a bowl.

7. Cover the bowl of marinade and refrigerate.

8. Arrange the steak onto a chopping board.

9. Place the tapenade onto the steak evenly and top with the spinach, followed by the feta cheese.

1. 10 Carefully roll the steak tightly to make a log.

10. With 6 kitchen string pieces, tie the log at 6 places.

11. Carefully cut the log between strings into 6 equal pieces, leaving string in place.

12. In a bowl, add the reserved marinade, tomatoes and salt and toss to coat.

13. Arrange the log pieces onto the prepared baking dish, cut-side up.

14. Now, arrange the tomatoes around the pinwheels evenly.

15. Bake for about 25-35 minutes.

16. Remove from the oven and put aside for about 5 minutes before serving.

Beef & Broccoli Bowl

Serving: 1

Preparation time: 15 minutes

Cooking time: 12 minutes

Ingredients:

- 4 ounces of lean ground beef
- 1 cup of broccoli, cut into bite-sized pieces
- 2 tablespoons of low-sodium chicken broth
- ¼ cup of tomatoes, chopped
- ¼ teaspoon of onion powder
- ¼ teaspoon of garlic powder
- Pinch of red pepper flakes
- Salt, to taste
- 1 ounce of low-fat cheddar cheese

Instructions:

1. Heat a lightly greased skillet over medium heat and cook the meat for about 8-10 minutes or until browned completely.

2. Meanwhile, in a microwave-safe bowl, place the broccoli and broth.
3. With a plastic wrap, cover the bowl and microwave for about 4 minutes.
4. Remove from the microwave and put aside.
5. Drain the grease from skillet.
6. Add the tomatoes, garlic powder, onion powder, red pepper flakes and salt and stir to mix well.
7. Add the broccoli and toss to coat well.
8. Remove from the heat and transfer the meat mixture into a serving bowl.
9. Top with cheddar and serve.

Beef Taco Bowl

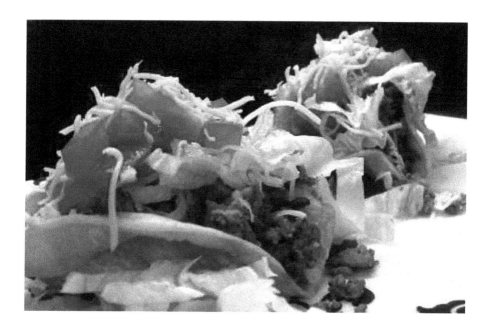

Servings: 4

Preparation time: 15 minutes

Cooking time: 15 minutes

Ingredients:

- 1 teaspoon of red chili powder
- 1 teaspoon of ground cumin
- Salt and freshly ground black pepper, to taste
- 1-pound flank steak, trimmed
- 2 scallions

- 1 lime, cut in half
- 8 cup of lettuce, torn
- 1 red bell pepper, seeded and sliced
- 1 cup of tomato, chopped
- ½ cup of fresh cilantro, chopped
- ¼ cup of light sour cream

Instructions:

1. Preheat the grill to medium-high heat. Grease the grill grate.
2. In a small bowl, mix together the spices, salt and black pepper.
3. Rub the steak with spice mixture generously.
4. Place the steak onto the grill and cook for about 4-6 minutes per side or until desired doneness.
5. Remove from the grill and place the steak onto a chopping board for about 5 minutes.
6. Now, place the scallions onto the grill and cook for about 1 minute per side.
7. Place the lime halves onto the grill, cut-side down and cook for about 1 minute.
8. Remove the scallions and lime halves from the grill and place onto a plate.
9. Chop the scallions roughly.
10. With a pointy knife, cut the steak into thin slices.

11. In a bowl, place the meat slices and chopped scallions.

12. Squeeze the lime halves over steak mixture and toss to coat well.

13. Divide lettuce into serving bowls and top each with bell pepper, followed by tomato, cilantro and beef mixture.

14. Top each bowl with soured cream and serve.

Veggie Stuffed Steak

Servings: 4

Preparation time: 15 minutes

Cooking time: 35 minutes

Ingredients:

- 1 (1½-pound) flank steak
- Salt and freshly ground black pepper, to taste
- 1 tablespoon of olive oil
- 2 small garlic cloves, minced
- 6 ounces of fresh spinach, chopped finely
- 1 medium green bell pepper, seeded and chopped
- 1 medium tomato, chopped finely

Instructions:

1. Preheat your oven to 425 degrees F. Grease a large baking dish.
2. Place beefsteak onto a flat surface.
3. Hold a pointy knife parallel to figure surface, slice the steak horizontally, without cutting all the way through, that you simply can open sort of a book.

4. With a meat mallet, flatten the steak to a good thickness. Sprinkle the steak with salt and black pepper evenly.

5. In a skillet, heat oil over medium heat and sauté garlic for about 1 minute.

6. Add spinach, with salt and black pepper and cook for about 2 minutes.

7. Stir in bell pepper and tomato and immediately remove from heat.

8. Transfer the spinach into a bowl and put aside to chill slightly.

9. Place the filling on the top of steak evenly.

10. Roll up the steak to seal the filling.

11. With cotton twine, tie the steak.

12. Place the steak roll into the prepared baking dish.

1. 13 Roast for about 30-35 minutes.

13. Remove from oven and let it cool slightly.

14. With a pointy knife, cut the roll into desired sized slices and serve.

Steak with Broccoli

Servings: 4

Preparation time: 15 minutes

Cooking time: 20 minutes

Ingredients:

- 16 ounces of sirloin steak, trimmed and cut into thin strips
- Salt and freshly ground black pepper, to taste
- 2 tablespoons of olive oil, divided
- 2 garlic cloves, minced
- 1 Serrano pepper, seeded and chopped finely
- 2 cups of broccoli florets
- 2 tablespoons of low-sodium soy sauce
- 2 tablespoons of fresh lime juice

Instructions:

1. Season the steak slices with black pepper.
2. Heat 1 tablespoon of oil in a large skillet over medium heat and cook the steak slices for about 6-8 minutes or until browned from all sides.

3. With a slotted spoon, transfer the steak slices onto a plate.
4. Heat remaining oil in the same skillet over medium heat and sauté the garlic and Serrano pepper for about 1 minute.
5. Add the broccoli and fry for about 2-3 minutes.
6. Stir in the cooked steak slices, soy and juice and cook for about 3-4 minutes.
7. Serve hot.

Beef with Mushrooms

Servings: 4

Preparation time: 15 minutes

Cooking time: 15 minutes

Ingredients:

For Beef:

- 4 (6-ounce of) beef tenderloin fillets
- Salt and freshly ground black pepper, to taste
- 2 tablespoons of olive oil, divided
- 1 teaspoon of garlic, smashed
- 1 tablespoon of fresh thyme, chopped

For Mushrooms:

- 2 tablespoons of olive oil
- 1-pound fresh mushrooms, sliced
- 2 teaspoons of garlic, smashed
- Salt and freshly ground black pepper, to taste

Instructions:

1. For beef: season the meat fillets with salt and black pepper evenly and put aside.
2. In a cast-iron skillet, heat the oil over medium heat and sauté the garlic and thyme for about 1 minute.
1. 3 Add the fillets and cook for about 5-7 minutes per side.
3. Meanwhile, for mushrooms: in another cast-iron skillet, heat the oil over medium heat and cook the mushrooms, garlic, salt, and black pepper for about 7-8 minutes, stirring frequently.
4. Divide the fillets onto serving plates.
5. Top with mushroom mixture and serve.

Steak with Carrot & Kale

Servings: 4

Preparation time: 15 minutes

Cooking time: 12 minutes

Ingredients:

- 2 tablespoons of olive oil
- 4 garlic cloves, minced
- 1-pound beef sirloin steak, cut into bite-sized pieces
- Freshly ground black pepper, to taste
- 1½ cups of carrots, peeled and cut into matchsticks
- 1½ cups of fresh kale, tough ribs removed and chopped
- 3 tablespoons of low-sodium soy sauce

Instructions:

1. In a skillet, heat the oil over medium heat and sauté the garlic for about 1 minute.
2. Add the meat and black pepper and stir to mix.
3. Increase the heat to medium-high and cook for about 3-4 minutes or until browned from all sides.

4. Add the carrot, kale and soy and cook for about 4-5 minutes.
5. Stir in the black pepper and take away from the heat.
6. Serve hot.

Ground Beef with Veggies

Servings: 4

Preparation time: 15 minutes

Cooking time: 25 minutes

Ingredients:

- 1-pound lean ground beef2 tablespoons of extra-virgin olive oil
- 2 garlic cloves, minced
- ½ of yellow onion, chopped
- 2 cups of fresh mushrooms, sliced
- 1 cup of fresh kale, tough ribs removed and chopped
- ¼ cup of low-sodium beef broth
- 2 tablespoons of balsamic vinegar
- 2 tablespoons of fresh parsley, chopped

Instructions:

1. Heat a large non-stick skillet over medium-high heat and cook the ground beef for about 8-10 minutes, ending the chunks with a wooden spoon.
2. With a slotted spoon, transfer the meat into a bowl.

3. In the same skillet, add the onion and garlic for about 3 minutes.

4. Add the mushrooms and cook for about 5-minutes.

5. Add the cooked beef, kale, broth and vinegar and bring to a boil.

6. Reduce the heat to medium-low and simmer for about 3 minutes.

1. 7 Stir in parsley and serve immediately.

Beef Chili

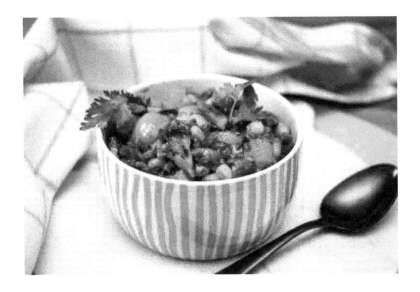

Servings: 8

Preparation time: 15 minutes

Cooking time: 1¾ hours

Ingredients:

- 2 tablespoons of olive oil
- 3 pounds ground beef
- 1 cup of yellow onion, chopped finely
- ½ cup of celery, chopped finely
- ½ cup of green bell pepper, seeded and chopped finely
- ½ cup of red bell pepper, seeded and chopped finely

- 1 (15-ounce of) can crushed tomatoes with juice
- 1½ cups of tomato juice
- 1½ teaspoons of Worcestershire sauce
- ½ teaspoon of dried oregano
- 3 tablespoons of red chili powder
- 1 teaspoon of ground cumin
- 1 teaspoon of garlic powder
- 1 teaspoon of salt
- ½ teaspoon of ground black pepper

Instructions:

1. In a large pan, heat the oil over medium-high heat and cook the meat for about 8-10 minutes or until browned.
2. Drain the grease from pan, leaving about 2 tablespoons inside.
3. In the pan, add the onions, celery and bell peppers over medium-high heat and cook for about 5 minutes, stirring frequently.
4. Add the tomatoes, tomato juice, Worcester sauce, oregano, spices, and stir to mix.
5. Reduce the heat to low and simmer, covered for about 1-1½ hours, stirring occasionally.
6. Serve hot.

Beef Stuffed Bell Peppers

Servings: 5

Preparation time: 20 minutes

Cooking time: 40 minutes

Ingredients:

- 5 large bell peppers, tops and seeds removed
- 1 tablespoon of olive oil
- ½ of large onion, chopped
- ½ teaspoon of dried oregano
- ½ teaspoon of dried thyme
- Salt and ground black pepper, as required
- 1-pound ground beef
- 1 large zucchini, chopped
- 3 tablespoons of homemade tomato paste

Instructions:

1. 1 Preheat your oven to 350 degrees F.
2. Grease a little baking dish.
3. In a large pan of the boiling water, place the bell peppers and cook for about 4-5 minutes.

4. Remove from the water and place onto a paper towel, cut side down.
5. Meanwhile, in a large nonstick wok, heat the vegetable oil over medium heat and sauté onion for about 3-4 minutes.
6. Add the ground beef, oregano, salt, and pepper and cook for about 8-10 minutes.
7. Add the zucchini and cook for about 2-3 minutes.
8. Remove from the heat and drain any juices from the meat mixture.
9. Add the ingredient and stir to mix.
10. Arrange the bell peppers into the prepared baking dish, cut side upward.
11. Stuff the bell peppers with the meat mixture evenly.
12. Bake for about 15 minutes.
13. Serve warm.

Garlicky Pork Tenderloin

Servings: 6

Preparation time: 10 minutes

Cooking time: 38 minutes

Ingredients:

- 3 medium garlic cloves, minced
- 3 teaspoons of dried rosemary, crushed
- ½ teaspoon of cayenne pepper
- Salt and ground black pepper, as required
- 2 pounds pork tenderloin
- 10 cups of fresh baby spinach

Instructions:

1. Preheat the oven to 400 degrees F.
2. Grease a roasting pan.
3. In a bowl, mix together all the Ingredients apart from pork and spinach.
4. Rub the pork with garlic mixture evenly.
5. Place the pork into prepared roasting pan.
6. Roast for about 25 minutes or until desired doneness.

7. Remove the roasting pan from oven and place the tenderloin onto a chopping board for about 10-15 minutes.

8. With a pointy knife, cut the tenderloin into desired size slices and serve alongside spinach.

Pork Stuffed Avocado

Servings: 8

Preparation time: 15 minutes

Cooking time: 10 minutes

Ingredients:

- 4 ripe avocados, halved and pitted
- 3 tablespoons of fresh lime juice
- 1 tablespoon of olive oil
- 1 medium onion, chopped
- 1-pound ground pork
- 1 packet taco seasoning
- Salt and ground black pepper, as required
- 2/3 cup of low-fat Mexican cheese, shredded
- ½ cup of lettuce, shredded
- ½ cup of cherry tomatoes, quartered

Instructions:

1. Carefully remove abut about 2-3 tablespoons of flesh from each avocado half.
2. Chop the avocado flesh and reserve it.

3. Arrange the avocado halves onto a tray and drizzle each with lime juice.
4. In a medium skillet, heat oil over medium heat and sauté the onion for about 5 minutes.
5. Add the ground pork, taco seasoning, salt and black pepper and cook for about 8-10 minutes, ending the meat with a wooden spoon.
6. Remove from the heat and drain the grease from the skillet.
7. Stuff each avocado half with pork and top with reserved avocado, cheese, lettuce and tomato.
8. Serve immediately.

Pork Burgers

Servings: 4

Preparation time: 15 minutes

Cooking time: 6 minutes

Ingredients:

For Patties:

- 1-pound lean ground pork
- ¼ cup of fresh parsley, chopped
- ¼ cup of fresh cilantro, chopped
- 1 tablespoon of fresh ginger, chopped
- 1 teaspoon of ground cumin
- 1 teaspoon of ground coriander
- ½ teaspoon of ground cinnamon
- Salt and ground black pepper, as required

For Salad:

- 6 cups of fresh baby arugula
- 2 cups of cherry tomatoes, quartered
- 1 tablespoon of fresh lemon juice
- 1 tablespoon of extra-virgin olive oil

Instructions:

1. In a bowl, add the pork, parsley, cilantro, ginger, spices, salt and black pepper and blend until well combined.
2. Make 4 equal-sized patties from the mixture.
3. Heat a greased grill pan over medium-high heat and cook the patties for about 3 minutes per side or until desired doneness.
4. Meanwhile, in a bowl, add arugula, tomatoes, juice, oil, and toss to coat well.
5. Divide the salad onto serving plates and top each with 1 patty.
6. Serve immediately.

Pork & Veggie Burgers

Servings: 4

Preparation time: 15 minutes

Cooking time: 16 minutes

Ingredients:

For Patties:

- 1-pound ground pork
- 1 carrot, peeled and chopped finely
- 1 medium raw beetroot, trimmed, peeled and chopped finely
- 1 small onion, chopped finely
- 2 Serrano peppers, seeded and chopped
- 1 tablespoon of fresh cilantro, chopped finely
- Salt and ground black pepper, as required
- 3 tablespoons of olive oil

For Burgers:

- 1 large onion, sliced
- 2 large tomatoes, sliced
- 4 lettuce leaves

Instructions:

1. For patties: in a large bowl, add all Ingredients apart from oil and blend until well combined.
2. Make equal-sized 8 patties from the mixture.
3. In a large non-stick sauté pan, heat the vegetable oil over medium heat and cook the patties in 2 batches for about 3-4 minutes per side or until golden brown.
4. Arrange the bun bottoms onto serving plates.
5. Plce1 patty over each bun, followed by the onion, tomato and lettuce.
6. Cover each with top of the bun and serve.

Rosemary Pork Tenderloin

Servings: 3

Preparation time: 10 minutes

Cooking time: 22 minutes

Ingredients:

- 1 teaspoon of fresh rosemary, minced
- 1 garlic clove, minced
- 1 tablespoon of fresh lemon juice
- 1 tablespoon of olive oil
- 1 teaspoon of Dijon mustard
- 1 teaspoon of powdered Erythritol
- Salt and ground black pepper, to taste
- 1-pound pork tenderloin
- 5 cups of fresh baby kale

Instructions:

1. Preheat your oven to 400 degrees F.
2. Grease a large rimmed baking sheet.
3. In a bowl, place all Ingredients except the tenderloin and cheese and beat until well combined.

4. Add tenderloin and coat with the mixture generously.

5. Arrange the tenderloin onto the prepared baking sheet.

6. Bake for about 20-22 minutes.

7. Remove baking sheet from the oven and place the tenderloin onto a chopping board for about 5 minutes.

8. With a pointy knife, cut the tenderloin into ¾-inch-thick slices and serve alongside the kale.

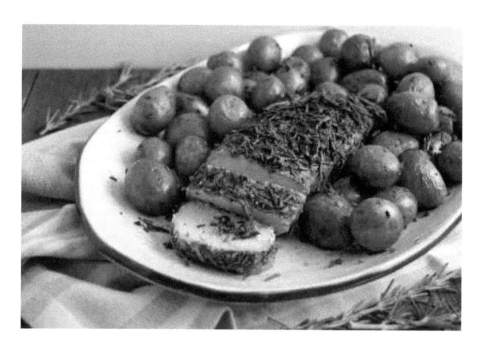

Pork with Veggies

Servings: 4

Preparation time: 15 minutes

Cooking time: 15 minutes

Ingredients:

- 1-pound pork loin, cut into thin strips
- 2 tablespoons of olive oil, divided
- 1 teaspoon of garlic, minced
- 1 teaspoon of fresh ginger, minced
- 2 tablespoons of low-sodium soy sauce
- 1 tablespoon of fresh lemon juice
- 1 tablespoon of Erythritol
- 1 teaspoon of arrowroot starch
- 10 ounces of broccoli florets
- 1 carrot, peeled and sliced
- 1 large red bell pepper, seeded and cut into strips
- 2 scallions, cut into 2-inch pieces

Instructions:

1. In a bowl, mix well pork strips, ½ tablespoon of olive oil, garlic, and ginger.
2. For sauce; add the soy sauce, lemon juice, Erythritol, and arrowroot starch in a small bowl and blend well.
3. Heat the remaining vegetable oil in a large nonstick skillet over high heat and sear the pork strips for about 3-4 minutes or until cooked through.
4. With a slotted spoon, transfer the pork into a bowl.
5. In the same skillet, add the carrot and cook for about 2-3 minutes.
6. Add the broccoli, bell pepper, and scallion and cook, covered for about 1-2 minutes.
7. Stir the cooked pork and sauce, and fry and cook for about 3-5 minutes or until the desired doneness, stirring occasionally.
8. Remove from the heat and serve.

Salmon Lettuce Wraps

Servings: 2

Preparation time: 10 minutes

Ingredients:

- ¼ cup of low-fat mozzarella cheese, cubed
- ¼ cup of tomato, chopped
- 2 tablespoons of fresh dill, chopped
- 1 teaspoon of fresh lemon juice
- Salt, as required
- 4 lettuce leaves
- 1/3 pound cooked salmon, chopped

Instructions:

1. In a small bowl, combine mozzarella, tomato, dill, lemon juice, and salt until well combined.
2. Arrange the lettuce leaves onto serving plates.
3. Divide the salmon and tomato mixture over each lettuce leaf and serve immediately.

Tuna Burgers

Servings: 2

Preparation time: 15 minutes

Cooking time: 6 minutes

Ingredients:

- 1 (15-ounce of) can water-packed tuna, drained
- ½ celery stalk, chopped
- 2 tablespoons of fresh parsley, chopped
- 1 teaspoon of fresh dill, chopped
- 2 tablespoon of walnuts, chopped
- 2 tablespoon of mayonnaise
- 1 egg, beaten
- 1 tablespoon of butter
- 3 cups of lettuce

Instructions:

1. For Burgers: add all Ingredients except the butter and lettuce in a bowl and blend until well combined.
2. Make 2 equal-sized patties from the mixture.

3. In a frying pan, melt butter over medium heat and cook the patties for about 2-3 minutes.
4. Carefully flip the side and cook for about 2-3 minutes.
5. Divide the lettuce onto serving plates.
6. Top each plate with 1 burger and serve.

Spicy Salmon

Servings: 4

Preparation time: 105 minutes

Cooking time: 8 minutes

Ingredients:

- 4 tablespoons of extra-virgin olive oil, divided
- 2 tablespoons of fresh lemon juice
- 1 teaspoon of ground turmeric
- 1 teaspoon of ground cumin
- Salt and ground black pepper, as required
- 4 (4-ounce of) boneless, skinless salmon fillets
- 6 cups of fresh arugula

Instructions:

1. In a bowl, mix together 2 tablespoons of oil, lemon juice, turmeric, cumin, salt and black pepper.
2. Add the salmon fillets and coat with the oil mixture generously. Set aside.
3. In a non-stick wok, heat remaining oil over medium heat.

4. Place salmon fillets, skin-side down and cook for about 3-5 minutes.
5. Change the side and cook for about 2-3 minutes more.
6. Divide the salmon onto serving plates and serve immediately alongside the arugula.

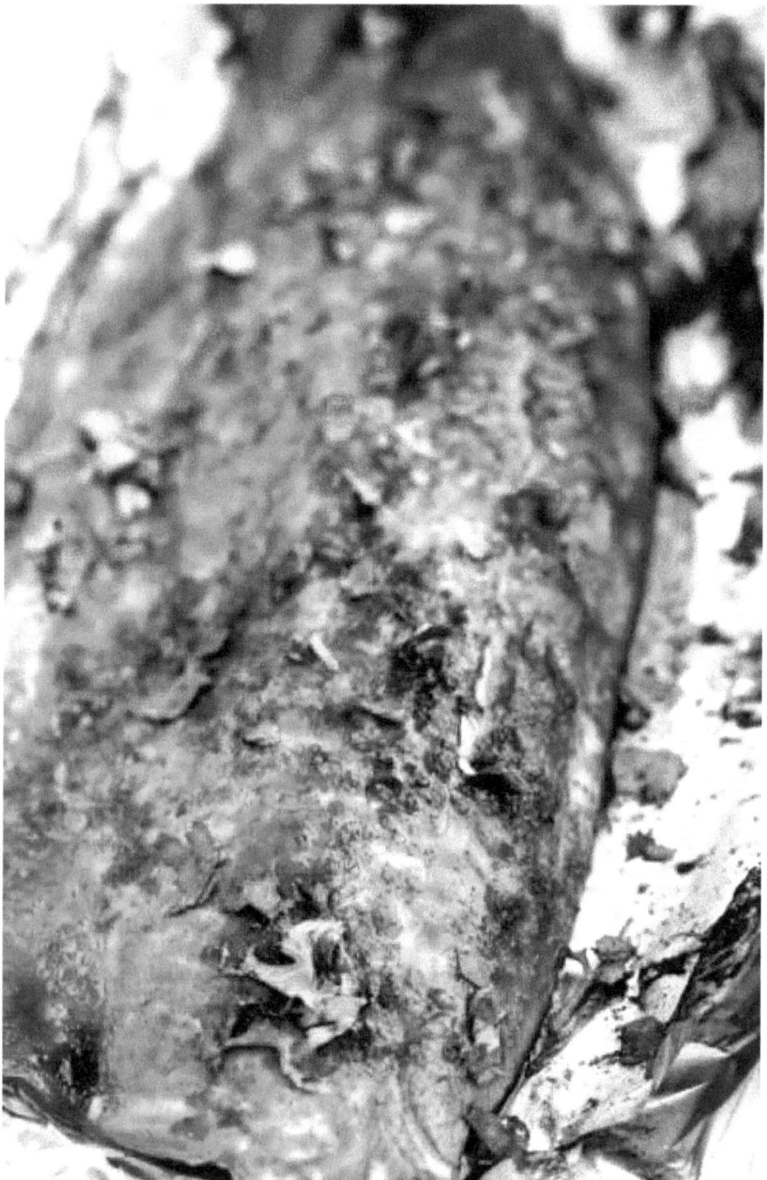

Lemony Salmon

Servings: 4

Preparation time: 10 minutes

Cooking time: 14 minutes

Ingredients:

- 2 garlic cloves, minced
- 1 tablespoon of fresh lemon zest, grated
- 2 tablespoon of olive oil
- 2 tablespoons of fresh lemon juice
- Salt and ground black pepper, to taste
- 4 (6-ounce of) boneless, skinless salmon fillets
- 6 cups of fresh spinach

Instructions:

1. Preheat the grill to medium-high heat.
2. Grease the grill grate.
3. In a bowl, place all Ingredients apart from salmon and spinach and blend well.
4. Add the salmon fillets and coat with garlic mixture generously.

5. Grill the salmon fillets for about 6-7 minutes per side.

6. Serve immediately alongside the spinach.

Zesty Salmon

Servings: 4

Preparation time: 10 minutes

Cooking time: 10 minutes

Ingredients:

- 1 tablespoon of butter, melted
- 1 tablespoon of fresh lemon juice 1 teaspoon of Worcestershire sauce
- 1 teaspoon of lemon zest, grated finely.
- 4 (6-ounce of) salmon fillets
- Salt and ground black pepper, to taste

Instructions:

1. In a baking dish, place butter, juice, Worcester sauce, and lemon peel, and blend well.
2. Coat the fillets with the mixture then arrange skin side-up in the baking dish.
3. Put aside for about 15 minutes.
4. Preheat the broiler of oven.
5. Arrange the oven rack about 6-inch from the element.

6. Line a broiler pan with a bit of foil.

7. Remove the salmon fillets from baking dish and season with salt and black pepper.

8. Arrange the salmon fillets onto the prepared broiler pan, skin side down.

9. Broil for about 8-10 minutes.

10. Serve hot.

Stuffed Salmon

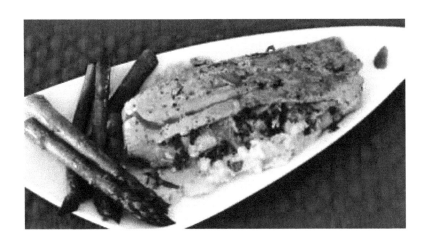

Servings: 4

Preparation time: 15 minutes

Cooking time: 16 minutes

Ingredients:

For Salmon:

- 4 (6-ounce of) skinless salmon fillets
- Salt and ground black pepper, as required
- 2 tablespoons of fresh lemon juice
- 2 tablespoons of olive oil, divided
- 1 tablespoon of unsalted butter

For Filling:

- 4 ounces of low-fat cream cheese, softened
- ¼ cup of low-fat Parmesan cheese, grated finely
- 4 ounces of frozen spinach, thawed and squeezed
- 2 teaspoons of garlic, minced
- Salt and ground black pepper, as required

Instructions:

1. Season each salmon fillet with salt and black pepper then, drizzle with lemon juice and 1 tablespoon of oil.
2. Arrange the salmon fillets onto a smooth surface.
3. With a pointy knife, cut a pocket into each salmon fillet about ¾ of the way through, being careful not to cut all the way.
4. For filling: In a bowl, add the cream cheese, Parmesan cheese, spinach, garlic, salt and black pepper and blend well.
5. Place about 1-2 tablespoons of spinach mixture into each salmon pocket and spread evenly.
6. In a skillet, heat the remaining oil and butter over medium-high heat and cook the salmon fillets for about 6-8 minutes per side.
7. Remove the salmon fillets from heat and transfer onto the serving plates.
8. Serve immediately.

Salmon with Asparagus

Servings: 6

Preparation time: 10 minutes

Cooking time: 20 minutes

Ingredients:

- 6 (4-ounce of) salmon fillets
- 2 tablespoons of extra-virgin olive oil
- 3 tablespoons of fresh parsley, minced
- ¼ teaspoon of ginger powder
- Salt and freshly ground black pepper, to taste
- 1½ pounds fresh asparagus

Instructions:

1. Preheat your oven to 400 degrees.
2. Grease a large baking dish.
3. In a bowl, place all Ingredients and blend well.
4. Arrange the salmon fillets into the prepared baking dish in a single layer.
5. Bake for about 15-20 minutes or until the desired doneness of salmon.

6. Meanwhile, in a pan of the boiling water, add asparagus and cook for about 4-5 minutes.
7. Drain the asparagus well.
8. Divide the asparagus onto serving plates evenly and top each with 1 salmon fillet and serve.

Salmon Parcel

Servings: 6

Preparation time: 15 minutes

Cooking time: 20 minutes

Ingredients:

- 6 (4-ounce of) salmon fillets
- Salt and freshly ground black pepper, to taste
- 1 yellow bell pepper, seeded and cubed
- 1 red bell pepper, seeded and cubed
- 4 plum tomatoes, cubed
- 1 small onion, sliced thinly
- ½ cup of fresh parsley, chopped
- ¼ cup of extra-virgin olive oil
- 2 tablespoons of fresh lemon juice

Instructions:

1. Preheat your oven to 400 degrees F.
2. Arrange 6 pieces of foil onto a smooth surface.
3. Place 1 salmon fillet on each bit of foil and sprinkle with salt and black pepper.

4. In a bowl, mix bell peppers, tomato and onion.
5. Place veggie mixture over each fillet evenly and top with parsley and capers evenly.
6. Drizzle with oil and lemon juice.
7. Fold each bit of foil around the salmon mixture to seal it.
8. Arrange the foil packets onto a large baking sheet in a single layer.
9. Bake for about 25 minutes.
10. Remove from the oven and place the foil packets onto serving plates.
11. Carefully unwrap each foil packet and serve.

Salmon with Cauliflower Mash

Servings: 4

Preparation time: 15 minutes

Cooking time: 20 minutes

Ingredients:

For Cauliflower Mash:

- 1-pound cauliflower, cut into florets
- 1 tablespoon of extra-virgin olive oil
- 3 garlic cloves, minced
- 1 teaspoon of fresh thyme leaves
- Salt and freshly ground black pepper, to taste

For Salmon:

- 1 (1-inch) piece fresh ginger, grated finely
- 1 tablespoon of honey
- 1 tablespoon of fresh lemon juice
- 1 tablespoon of Dijon mustard
- 2 tablespoons of olive oil
- 4 (6-ounce of) salmon fillets
- 2 tablespoons of fresh parsley, chopped

Instructions:

1. For mash: In a large saucepan of water, arrange a steamer basket and bring to a boil.
2. Place the cauliflower florets in a steamer basket and steam covered for about 10 minutes.
3. Drain the cauliflower and put aside.
4. In a small frying pan, heat the oil over medium heat and sauté the garlic for about 2 minutes.
5. Remove the frying pan from heat and transfer the garlic oil in a large food processor.
6. Add the cauliflower, thyme, salt and black pepper and pulse until smooth.
7. Transfer the cauliflower mash into a bowl and put aside.
8. Meanwhile, in a bowl, mix ginger, honey, juice and Dijon mustard. Set aside.
9. In a large non-stick skillet, heat vegetable oil over medium-high heat and cook the salmon fillets for about 3-4 minutes per side.
10. Stir in honey mixture and immediately remove from heat.
11. Divide warm cauliflower mash onto serving plates.
12. Top each plate with 1 salmon fillet and serve.

Salmon with Salsa

Servings: 4

Preparation time: 15 minutes

Cooking time: 8 minutes

Ingredients:

For Salsa:

- 2 large ripe avocados, peeled, pitted and cut into small chunks
- 1 small tomato, chopped
- 2 tablespoons of red onion, chopped finely
- ¼ cup of fresh cilantro, chopped finely
- 1 tablespoon of jalapeño pepper, seeded and minced finely
- 1 garlic clove, minced finely
- 3 tablespoon of fresh lime juice
- Salt and ground black pepper, as required

For Salmon:

- 4 (5-ounce of) (1-inch thick) salmon fillets
- Sea salt and ground black pepper, as required
- 3 tablespoons of olive oil

- 1 tablespoon of fresh rosemary leaves, chopped
- 1 tablespoon of fresh lemon juice

Instructions:

1. For salsa: add all Ingredients in a bowl and gently, stir to mix.
2. With a plastic wrap, cover the bowl and refrigerate before serving.
3. For salmon: season each salmon fillet with salt and black pepper generously.
4. In a large skillet, heat the oil over medium-high heat.
5. Place the salmon fillets, skins side up and cook for about 4 minutes.
6. Carefully change the side of every salmon fillet and cook for about 4 minutes more.
7. Stir in the rosemary and juice and take away from the heat.
8. Divide the salsa onto serving plates evenly.
9. to every plate with 1 salmon fillet and serve.

Walnut Crusted Salmon

Servings: 2

Preparation time: 15 minutes

Cooking time: 20 minutes

Ingredients:

- ½ cup of walnuts
- 1 tablespoon of fresh dill, chopped
- 2 tablespoons of fresh lemon rind, grated
- Salt and ground black pepper, as required
- 1 tablespoon of coconut oil, melted
- 3-4 tablespoons of Dijon mustard
- 4 (3-ounce of) salmon fillets
- 4 teaspoons of fresh lemon juice
- 3 cups of fresh baby spinach

Instructions:

1. Preheat your oven to 350 degrees F.
2. Line a large baking sheet with parchment paper.
3. Place the walnuts in a food processor and pulse until chopped roughly.

4. Add the dill, lemon peel, garlic salt, black pepper, butter, and pulse until a crumbly mixture forms.
5. Place the salmon fillets onto the prepared baking sheet in a single layer, skin-side down.
6. Coat the top of every salmon fillet with Dijon mustard.
7. Place the walnut mixture over each fillet and gently, press into the surface of salmon.
8. Bake for about 15–20 minutes.
9. Remove the salmon fillets from the oven and transfer onto the serving plates.
10. Drizzle with the juice and serve alongside the spinach.

Garlicky Tilapia

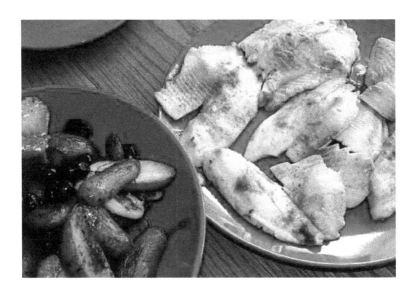

Servings: 4

Preparation time: 10 minutes

Cooking time: 5 minutes

Ingredients:

- 2 tablespoons of olive oil
- 4 (5-ounce of) tilapia fillets
- 3 garlic cloves, minced
- 1 tablespoon of fresh ginger, minced
- 2-3 tablespoons of low-sodium chicken broth
- Salt and ground black pepper, to taste

- 6 cups of fresh baby spinach

Instructions:

1. In a large sauté pan, heat the oil over medium heat and cook the tilapia fillets for about 3 minutes.
2. Flip the side and stir in the garlic and ginger.
3. Cook for about 1-2 minutes.
4. Add the broth and cook for about 2-3 more minutes.
5. Stir in salt and black pepper and take away from heat.
6. Serve hot alongside the spinach.

Tilapia Piccata

Servings: 4

Preparation time: 15 minutes

Cooking time: 8 minutes

Ingredients:

- 3 tablespoons of fresh lemon juice
- 2 tablespoons of olive oil
- 2 garlic cloves, minced
- ½ teaspoon of lemon zest, grated
- 2 teaspoons of capers, drained
- 2 tablespoons of fresh basil, minced
- 4 (6-ounce of) tilapia fillets
- Salt and ground black pepper, as required
- 6 cups of fresh baby kale

Instructions:

1. Preheat the broiler of the oven.
2. Arrange an oven rack about 4-inch from the heating element.
3. Grease a broiler pan.

4. In a small bowl, add the lemon juice, oil, garlic and lemon peel and beat until well combined.
5. Add the capers and basil and stir to mix.
6. Reserve 2 tablespoons of mixture in a small bowl.
7. Coat the fish fillets with remaining capers mixture and sprinkle with salt and black pepper.
8. Place the tilapia fillets onto the broiler pan and broil for about 3-4 minutes side.
9. Remove from the oven and place the fish fillets onto serving plates.
10. Drizzle with reserved capers mixture and serve alongside the kale.

Cod in Dill Sauce

Servings: 2

Preparation time: 10 minutes

Cooking time: 13 minutes

Ingredients:

- 2 (6-ounce of) cod fillets
- 1 teaspoon of onion powder
- Salt and ground black pepper, as required
- 3 tablespoons of butter, divided
- 2 garlic cloves, minced
- 1-2 lemon slices
- 2 teaspoons of fresh dill weed
- 3 cups of fresh spinach, torn

Instructions:

1. Season each cod fillet evenly with the onion powder, salt and black pepper.
2. In a medium skillet, heat 1 tablespoon of oil over high heat and cook the cod fillets for about 4-5 minutes per side.

3. Transfer the cod fillets onto a plate.

4. Meanwhile, in a frying pan, heat the remaining oil over low heat and sauté the garlic and lemon slices for about 40-60 seconds.

5. Stir in the cooked cod fillets and dill and cook, covered for about 1-2 minutes.

6. Remove the cod fillets from heat and transfer onto the serving plates.

7. Top with the pan sauce and serve immediately alongside the spinach.

Cod & Veggies Bake

Servings: 4

Preparation time: 15 minutes

Cooking time: 20 minutes

Ingredients:

- 1 teaspoon of olive oil
- ½ cup of onion, minced
- 1 cup of zucchini, chopped
- 1 garlic clove, minced
- 2 tablespoons of fresh basil, chopped
- 2 cups of fresh tomatoes, chopped
- Salt and ground black pepper, as required
- 4 (6-ounce of) cod steaks
- 1/3 cup of feta cheese, crumbled

Instructions:

1. Preheat your oven to 450 degrees F.
2. Grease a large shallow baking dish.
3. In a skillet, heat oil over medium heat and sauté the onion, zucchini and garlic for about 4-5 minutes.

4. Stir in the basil, tomatoes, salt and black pepper and immediately remove from heat.
5. Place the cod steaks into the prepared baking dish in a single layer and top with tomato mixture evenly.
6. Sprinkle with the cheese evenly.
7. Bake for about 15 minutes or until desired doneness.
8. Serve hot.

Cod & Veggie Pizza

Servings: 3

Preparation time: 20 minutes

Cooking time: 1 hour

Ingredients:

For Base:

- Olive oil cooking spray
- ¼ cup of oat flour
- 2 teaspoons of dried rosemary, crushed
- Freshly ground black pepper, to taste
- 4 egg whites
- 2½ teaspoons of olive oil
- ½ cup of low-fat Parmesan cheese, grated freshly
- 2 cups of zucchini, grated and squeezed

For Topping:

- 1 cup of tomato paste
- 1 teaspoon of fresh rosemary, minced
- 1 teaspoon of fresh basil, minced
- Freshly ground black pepper, to taste

- 4 cups of fresh mushrooms, chopped
- 1 tomato, chopped
- 3 ounces of boneless cod fillet, chopped
- 1½ cups of onion, sliced into rings
- 1 red bell pepper, seeded and chopped
- 1 green bell pepper, seeded and chopped
- 1/3 cup of low-fat mozzarella, shredded

Instructions:

1. Preheat your oven to 400 degrees F.
2. Grease a pie dish with cooking spray.
3. For base: in a large bowl, add all the Ingredients and blend until well combined.
4. Transfer the mixture into the prepared pie dish and press to smooth the surface.
5. Bake for about 40 minutes.
6. Remove from the oven and put aside to chill for at least 15 minutes.
7. Carefully end up the crust onto a baking sheet.
8. For topping: in a bowl, add tomato paste, herbs and black pepper.
9. Spread spaghetti sauce mixture over the crust evenly.
10. Arrange the vegetables over spaghetti sauce, followed by the cheese.
11. Bake for about 20 minutes or until cheese is melted.

12. Serve hot.

Garlicky Haddock

Servings: 2

Preparation time: 10 minutes

Cooking time: 11 minutes

Ingredients:

- 2 tablespoons of olive oil, divided
- 4 garlic cloves, minced and divided
- 1 teaspoon of fresh ginger, grated finely
- 2 (4-ounce of) haddock fillets
- Salt and freshly ground black pepper, to taste
- 3 cup of fresh baby spinach

Instructions:

1. In a skillet, heat 1 tablespoon of oil over medium heat and sauté 2 garlic cloves and ginger for about 1 minute.
2. Add the haddock fillets, salt and black pepper and cook for about 3-5 minutes per side or until desired doneness.
3. Meanwhile, in another skillet, heat remaining oil over medium heat and heat and sauté remaining garlic for about 1 minute.

4. Add the spinach, salt and black pepper and cook for about 4-5 minutes.
5. Divide the spinach onto serving plates and top each with 1 haddock fillet.
6. Serve immediately.

Haddock in Parsley Sauce

Servings: 2

Preparation time: 10 minutes

Cooking time: 9 minutes

Ingredients:

- 2 (5-ounce of) haddock fillets
- Salt and ground black pepper, as required
- 2 tablespoons of olive oil
- 1 tablespoon of fresh parsley, chopped
- 1 tablespoon of fresh lime juice
- 3 cups of fresh arugula

Instructions:

1. In a large skillet, heat the oil over medium-high heat.
2. Place the haddock fillets, skins side up and cook for about 4 minutes.
3. Carefully change the side of every fillet and cook for about 4 minutes more.
4. Stir in the parsley and juice and take away from the heat.
5. Serve hot alongside the arugula.

Halibut with Zucchini

Servings: 4

Preparation time: 15 minutes

Cooking time: 20 minutes

Ingredients:

- 1 teaspoon of olive oil
- ½ cup of yellow onion, minced
- 1 cup of zucchini, chopped
- 2 garlic cloves, minced
- 2 tablespoons of fresh basil, chopped
- 2 cups of fresh tomatoes, chopped
- Salt and freshly ground black pepper, to taste
- 4 (6-ounce) of halibut steaks
- 1/3 cup of feta cheese, crumbled

Instructions:

1. Preheat your oven to 450 degrees F.
2. Grease a large shallow baking dish.
3. In a skillet, heat the oil over medium heat and sauté the onion, zucchini and garlic for about 4-5 minutes.

4. Stir in the basil, tomatoes and black pepper and immediately remove from heat.
5. Place the halibut steaks into the prepared baking dish in a single layer.
6. Top with the tomato mixture evenly and sprinkle with cheese evenly.
7. Bake for about 15 minutes or until desired doneness.
8. Serve hot.

Roasted Mackerel

Servings: 2

Preparation time: 10 minutes

Cooking time: 20 minutes

Ingredients:

- 2 (7-ounce of) mackerel fillets
- 1 tablespoon of olive oil
- Salt and ground black pepper, to taste
- 3 cups of fresh baby greens

Instructions:

1. Preheat your oven to 350 degrees F.
2. Arrange a rack in the middle of the oven.
3. Lightly grease a baking dish.
4. Brush the fish fillets with melted butter then season with salt and black pepper.
5. Arrange the fish fillets into the prepared baking dish in a single layer.
6. Bake for about 20 minutes.
7. Serve hot alongside the greens.

Herbed Sea Bass

Servings: 2

Preparation time: 10 minutes

Cooking time: 20 minutes

Ingredients:

- 2 (1¼-pound) whole sea bass, gutted, gilled, scaled and fins removed
- Salt and ground black pepper, as required
- 6 fresh bay leaves
- 2 fresh thyme sprigs
- 2 fresh parsley sprigs
- 2 fresh rosemary sprigs
- 2 tablespoons of butter, melted
- 2 tablespoons of fresh lemon juice
- 3 cups of fresh arugula

Instructions:

1. Season the cavity and outer side of every fish with salt and black pepper evenly.

2. With a plastic wrap, cover each fish and refrigerate for 1 hour.
3. Preheat the oven to 450 degrees F.
4. Lightly grease a baking dish.
5. Arrange 2 bay leaves in the bottom of the prepared baking dish.
6. Divide herb sprigs and remaining bay leaves inside the cavity of every fish.
7. Arrange both fish over bay leave in the baking dish and drizzle with butter.
8. Roast for about 15-20 minutes or until fish is cooked through.
9. Remove the baking dish from oven and place the fish onto a platter.
10. Drizzle the fish with juice and serve alongside the arugula.

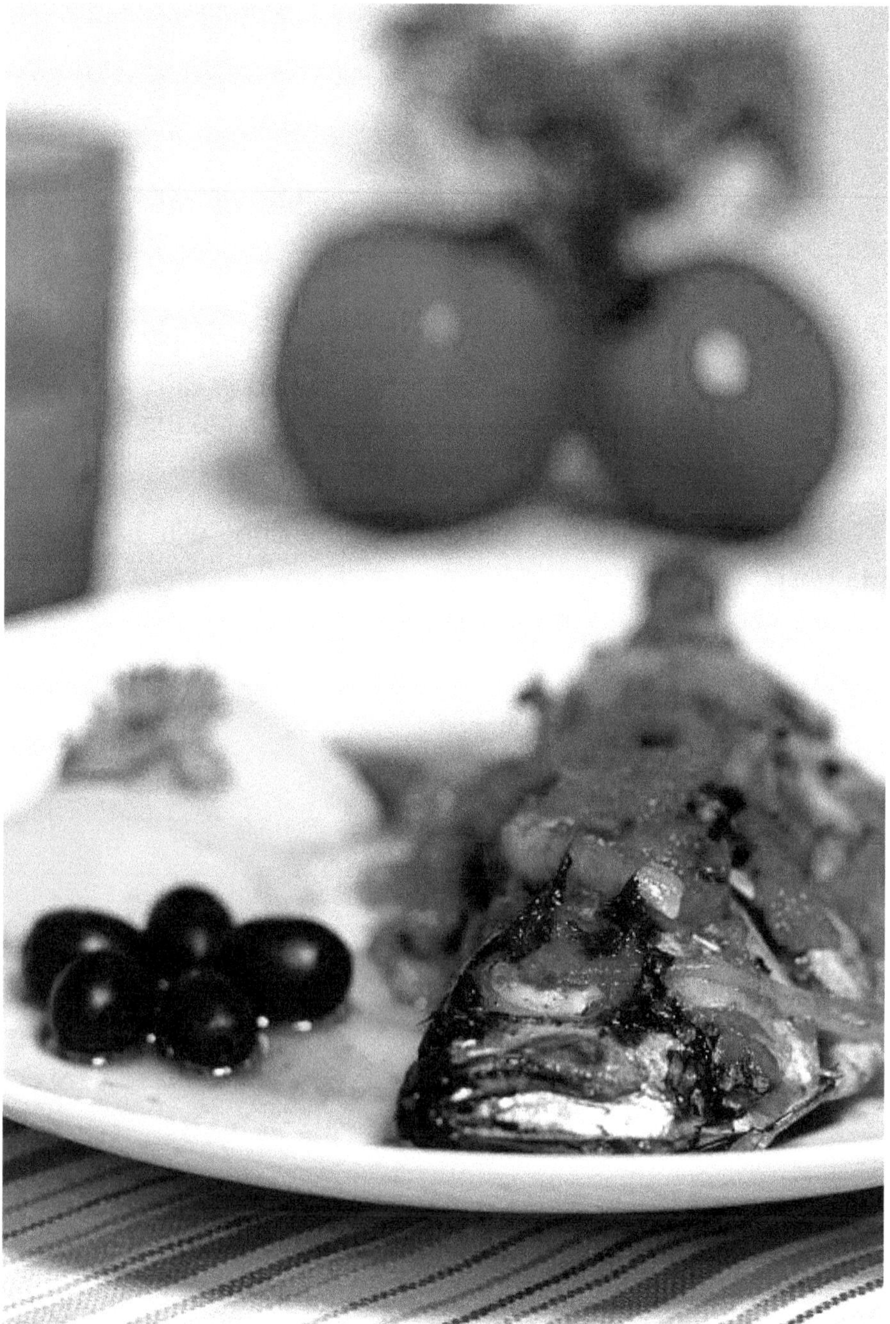

Lightning Source UK Ltd.
Milton Keynes UK
UKHW020729210621
385887UK00005B/175